WOMEN HEALTH CHALLENGES AGE 70

Empowering Wellness and Vitality in Your Golden Years

Becky Morgan

DEDICATION

To all the remarkable women over 70,

Your strength, wisdom, and resilience inspire us every day. This book is dedicated to your journey of health and well-being. May it guide you in embracing your golden years with confidence and joy.

With admiration and gratitude,

Becky Morgan.

TABLE OF CONTENTS

DEDICATION...2

INTRODUCTION...5

Welcome to Your Golden Years..........................5

Embracing Health and Wellness.......................8

How to Use This Book....................................9

PART I..12

UNDERSTANDING HEALTH CHANGES AT AGE 70..12

CHAPTER 1: THE AGING PROCESS..........14

CHAPTER 2: COMMON HEALTH CHALLENGES FOR WOMEN OVER 70.....20

PART II:..28

PHYSICAL HEALTH AND MOBILITY.......28

CHAPTER 3: MAINTAINING MOBILITY AND PHYSICAL ACTIVITY......................30

Importance of Staying Active...........................30

Low-Impact Exercises and Routines...............31

Tips for Enhancing Mobility...........................33

CHAPTER 4: BONE HEALTH AND OSTEOPOROSIS.......................................38

Understanding Bone Density Loss...................38

Preventing and Managing Osteoporosis..........39

Dietary and Lifestyle Recommendations..........41

PART III:..46

CARDIOVASCULAR AND CHRONIC HEALTH..46

CHAPTER 5: CARDIOVASCULAR HEALTH..48

Heart Disease in Women Over 70...................48

Preventive Measures and Screenings................50

Heart-Healthy Diet and Lifestyle....................52

CHAPTER 6: MANAGING CHRONIC CONDITIONS................................56

Diabetes: Prevention and Control....................56

Hypertension: Monitoring and Management..59

Arthritis: Types, Pain Management, and Physical Therapy.................................62

PART IV:.................................65

COGNITIVE AND MENTAL HEALTH........65

CHAPTER 7: COGNITIVE HEALTH AND DEMENTIA.................................67

Understanding Cognitive Decline....................67

Early Signs of Dementia.................................68

Strategies for Maintaining Cognitive Function 70

CHAPTER 8: MENTAL HEALTH AND EMOTIONAL WELL-BEING......................75

Recognizing Depression and Anxiety..............75

Coping Mechanisms and Support Systems......77

The Importance of Social Connections...........80

CHAPTER 9: NUTRITIONAL NEEDS FOR WOMEN OVER 70....................................83

Key Nutrients for Aging Gracefully.................83

Dietary Recommendations and Meal Plans.....86

Supplements and Their Role...........................88

CHAPTER 10: CANCER SCREENING AND PREVENTION................................92

Common Cancers in Women Over 70..............92

Recommended Screenings and Tests...............94

Lifestyle Choices for Cancer Prevention..........97

CHAPTER 11: REGULAR HEALTH CHECK-UPS 102

Importance of Routine Check-Ups 102

What to Expect During Health Appointments 104

Building a Relationship with Your Healthcare Provider 108

CONCLUSION: EMBRACING YOUR GOLDEN YEARS 113

Recap of Key Points 113

Staying Motivated and Positive 116

BONUS CHAPTER 120

Sample Meal Plans and Recipes 120

Nutritious and Easy-to-Prepare Recipes 121

Quinoa and Vegetable Stir-Fry 121

Baked Salmon with Lemon and Dill 124

Spinach and Chickpea Salad 127

Turkey and Avocado Wrap 130

Lentil and Vegetable Soup 132

Meal Plans for Different Dietary Needs 135

Heart-Healthy Meal Plan 135

Diabetic-Friendly Meal Plan 135

Bone Health Meal Plan 136

Anti-Inflammatory Meal Plan 137

INTRODUCTION

Welcome to Your Golden Years

A Life of Inspiration: My Grandma, Agnes

My grandma, Agnes, is an inspiration to our entire family. At 72 years old, she remains energetic, fit, and strong. While many women her age face health challenges like osteoporosis, frailty, and cognitive decline, Agnes has defied the odds.

Agnes credits her health to a lifetime of healthy habits. She exercises daily, enjoying brisk walks and yoga sessions. Social connections are a priority for her; she volunteers at local charities and often meets friends for tea, keeping her social calendar as active as her physical routine.

Her diet is a model of balance and nutrition. Rich in fruits, vegetables, whole grains, and lean proteins, Agnes avoids processed foods and sugars. Instead, she embraces natural remedies like turmeric and ginger to manage joint pain and inflammation.

Despite some memory loss, she stays mentally active by engaging in reading, puzzles, and learning new skills such as painting and cooking. Her positive attitude and strong faith also play a significant role in her overall well-being.

My grandma's story shows that with determination, healthy choices, and a supportive community, women can thrive even in their 70s. She inspires us all to prioritize our health and embrace aging with grace and vitality.

The Journey to 70 and Beyond

Reaching 70 is a significant milestone, one that reflects a life rich with experiences, wisdom, and growth. It's a journey that has seen us navigate various life stages, from youth and adulthood to middle age and now senior years. Each stage has brought its own set of challenges and triumphs, shaping us into who we are today.

At 70, it's natural to reflect on the past while looking forward to the future. This period offers a chance to embrace new hobbies, reconnect with loved ones, and focus on what truly matters. It's also a time to prioritize our health and well-being, ensuring that we can enjoy this phase of life to its fullest.

Embracing Health and Wellness

Maintaining good health is crucial at any age, but it becomes especially important as we grow older. Our bodies and minds undergo various changes, and staying proactive about our health can make a significant difference in our quality of life.

Embracing health and wellness means adopting habits that support our physical, mental, and emotional well-being. This includes regular physical activity, a balanced diet, and routine medical check-ups. It also involves nurturing our mental health by staying socially active, engaging in stimulating activities, and seeking support when needed.

It's important to remember that wellness is a holistic concept. It encompasses not only our physical health but also our mental and emotional states. Finding a balance that works for us individually is key to living a fulfilling and vibrant life.

How to Use This Book

This book is designed to be a comprehensive guide for women in their 70s, addressing the unique health challenges and opportunities that come with this stage of life. Whether you're looking for advice on managing chronic conditions, tips for staying active, or ways to enhance your mental well-being, you'll find valuable information within these pages.

Each chapter focuses on a specific aspect of health and wellness, providing detailed explanations, practical tips, and actionable advice. The goal is to empower you with the knowledge and tools needed to make informed decisions about your health and lifestyle.

As you read through the book, feel free to skip to the sections that are most relevant to you. There's no need to read it cover to cover unless you want to. The book is structured to allow you to find the information you need easily and quickly.

This book is more than just a collection of health tips. It's a companion that understands the unique joys and challenges of life at 70 and beyond. It's written with compassion and a deep understanding of what it means to navigate this stage of life. As you embark on this journey, know that you're not alone. We're here to support you every step of the way.

PART I

UNDERSTANDING HEALTH CHANGES AT AGE 70

CHAPTER 1: THE AGING PROCESS

Physical Changes

One of the most noticeable aspects of aging is the physical changes our bodies undergo. These changes are a natural part of the aging process and vary from person to person. Common physical changes include a decrease in muscle mass and strength, which can affect our ability to perform everyday tasks. It's essential to stay active and engage in regular exercise, such as walking, swimming, or light weightlifting, to maintain muscle strength and flexibility.

Bone density also tends to decrease with age, increasing the risk of fractures and osteoporosis. Ensuring adequate calcium and vitamin D intake, either through diet or supplements, can help maintain bone health. Weight-bearing exercises, like walking or resistance training, are beneficial in strengthening bones and reducing the risk of osteoporosis.

Our skin changes as well, becoming thinner and less elastic. This can lead to wrinkles, dryness, and an increased susceptibility to bruises and cuts. It's important to keep the skin hydrated by using moisturizers and drinking plenty of water. Protecting your skin from the sun by wearing sunscreen and protective clothing can also prevent damage.

Another significant change is the slowing of metabolism, which can lead to weight gain if dietary habits remain the same. It's crucial to adopt a balanced diet rich in fruits, vegetables, whole grains, and lean proteins while reducing the intake of processed foods and sugars. Staying physically active can also help manage weight and promote overall health.

Vision and hearing might also decline. Regular eye exams can help detect issues like cataracts or glaucoma early on, while hearing tests can address hearing loss. Using glasses, hearing aids, or other assistive devices can significantly improve quality of life.

Mental and Cognitive Changes

Aging also brings about changes in our mental and cognitive functions. It's common to experience some degree of memory loss or slower cognitive processing as we age. However, these changes do not necessarily mean a decline in overall mental capabilities.

Staying mentally active is crucial in maintaining cognitive health. Engaging in activities that stimulate the brain, such as puzzles, reading, learning new skills, or playing musical instruments, can help keep the mind sharp. Social interactions are equally important; maintaining relationships with family and friends can provide emotional support and mental stimulation.

It's also beneficial to establish routines that incorporate mental exercises. Regularly practicing mindfulness or meditation can improve focus and cognitive function. Additionally, ensuring adequate sleep is vital for cognitive health, as the brain uses this time to consolidate memories and repair itself.

It's important to distinguish between normal age-related cognitive changes and more serious conditions like dementia or Alzheimer's disease. If you notice significant memory loss, confusion, or changes in personality, it's essential to consult a healthcare professional for a thorough evaluation.

Emotional Well-being

Emotional well-being is an integral part of overall health, especially as we age. Many people experience a range of emotions as they navigate the later stages of life, including happiness, satisfaction, anxiety, and sometimes sadness. It's normal to reflect on past experiences and contemplate the future.

Maintaining a positive outlook can greatly influence emotional health. Finding joy in everyday activities, whether it's spending time with loved ones, pursuing hobbies, or volunteering, can provide a sense of purpose and fulfillment. Engaging in social activities and staying connected with friends and family can also alleviate feelings of loneliness and isolation.

It's not uncommon to experience grief or sadness, particularly if dealing with the loss of loved ones or significant life changes. Seeking support from friends, family, or support groups can be incredibly helpful. In some cases, talking to a mental health professional can provide the necessary tools and strategies to manage these emotions.

Practicing self-compassion is equally important. Aging is a natural process, and it's essential to be kind to oneself during this time. Acknowledge your feelings, celebrate your achievements, and accept the changes that come with age.

Incorporating relaxation techniques into your daily routine can also enhance emotional well-being. Activities such as yoga, meditation, and deep breathing exercises can reduce stress and promote a sense of calm.

By understanding and addressing the physical, mental, and emotional changes that come with aging, we can take proactive steps to maintain our health and well-being. This holistic approach ensures that we not only live longer but also enjoy a higher quality of life in our golden years.

CHAPTER 2: COMMON HEALTH CHALLENGES FOR WOMEN OVER 70

Women over 70 often face several key health concerns. One prevalent issue is cardiovascular health. Heart disease is a leading cause of death among older adults. With age, blood vessels and arteries become less flexible, leading to hypertension and increasing the risk of heart attacks and strokes. Regular physical activity, a balanced diet low in saturated fats and high in fruits and vegetables, and regular check-ups with a healthcare provider can help manage and reduce these risks. Blood pressure and cholesterol levels should be monitored regularly to detect any issues early.

Bone health is another critical concern. Osteoporosis, a condition where bones become brittle and fragile, is common among older women due to the decrease in estrogen levels after menopause. This makes bones more susceptible to fractures.

Ensuring adequate calcium and vitamin D intake, along with weight-bearing exercises like walking or resistance training, can help maintain bone density. Bone density tests are recommended to monitor bone health and take necessary measures if needed.

Cognitive health is also a significant area of focus. Many women over 70 worry about memory loss and cognitive decline, which can be early signs of dementia or Alzheimer's disease. Mental exercises, such as puzzles, reading, and learning new skills, can help keep the brain active. Social engagement and staying connected with family and friends are crucial for mental well-being. It's important to distinguish normal age-related memory changes from more serious cognitive impairments, and consult a healthcare professional if there are concerns.

Vision and hearing often decline with age, impacting daily life and independence. Regular eye exams are essential to detect conditions like cataracts, glaucoma, or macular degeneration early. Hearing loss can be managed with hearing aids or other assistive devices. Addressing these sensory changes promptly can greatly improve quality of life.

Managing chronic conditions becomes increasingly important as we age. Conditions such as diabetes, hypertension, and arthritis are common among women over 70. These conditions require regular monitoring and management to prevent complications. A balanced diet, regular physical activity, and adherence to prescribed medications are vital. Working closely with healthcare providers to manage these conditions can help maintain health and prevent complications.

Mental health is another crucial aspect of overall well-being. Older adults may experience depression or anxiety due to various factors, including health problems, loss of loved ones, or social isolation. Staying socially active, participating in community activities, and seeking support from friends, family, or mental health professionals can help manage these feelings. Mindfulness practices, such as meditation or yoga, can also promote emotional well-being.

Maintaining a healthy weight can become more challenging with age due to a slower metabolism and decreased physical activity. Being overweight or underweight can both pose health risks. A balanced diet rich in nutrients and regular physical activity can help manage weight effectively. Consulting with a nutritionist or dietitian can provide personalized dietary advice to meet specific needs.

Skin health is another area that requires attention. Aging skin becomes thinner, less elastic, and more prone to bruises and cuts. Proper skin care, including regular moisturizing and protection from excessive sun exposure, is essential. Using sunscreen and wearing protective clothing can prevent skin damage and reduce the risk of skin cancer.

Urinary health can also be a concern for older women. Issues such as urinary incontinence or frequent urinary tract infections are common. Pelvic floor exercises, such as Kegel exercises, can help strengthen the muscles that control urination. Staying hydrated, practicing good hygiene, and consulting a healthcare provider if problems persist are important steps in managing urinary health.

Sleep patterns often change with age, and many older adults experience difficulties with sleep. Poor sleep can affect overall health and well-being. Establishing a regular sleep routine, creating a comfortable sleep environment, and avoiding caffeine or heavy meals before bedtime can improve sleep quality. If sleep problems persist, it's important to seek advice from a healthcare provider.

Preventive care and regular health screenings are essential for women over 70. Regular check-ups with a healthcare provider can help monitor health conditions, update vaccinations, and conduct screenings for various cancers, such as breast, colorectal, and cervical cancer.

Early detection of health issues can lead to more effective treatment and better outcomes.

It's also important to stay physically active. Regular exercise can help maintain mobility, strength, and balance, reducing the risk of falls and improving overall health. Activities like walking, swimming, tai chi, or yoga are excellent for maintaining physical fitness and flexibility. Exercise also has mental health benefits, helping to reduce stress and anxiety.

Nutrition plays a vital role in maintaining health. A balanced diet that includes a variety of fruits, vegetables, whole grains, lean proteins, and healthy fats is essential. Adequate hydration is equally important. Nutritional needs may change with age, and it may be necessary to adjust the diet to ensure proper nutrient intake. Supplements can be used if needed, but it's best to obtain nutrients from a well-rounded diet.

Staying mentally active and engaged is crucial for cognitive health. Activities that stimulate the mind, such as reading, puzzles, or engaging in hobbies, can help keep the brain sharp. Social interactions and meaningful relationships also play a significant role in mental well-being. Joining clubs, volunteering, or participating in community activities can provide opportunities for social engagement.

27

PART II:

PHYSICAL HEALTH AND MOBILITY

CHAPTER 3:
MAINTAINING MOBILITY AND PHYSICAL ACTIVITY

Importance of Staying Active

Staying active is crucial for maintaining overall health and preventing a range of health issues. Regular physical activity helps to maintain muscle strength, bone density, and joint flexibility. It also supports cardiovascular health, helping to control blood pressure, improve circulation, and reduce the risk of heart disease and stroke.

Physical activity plays a vital role in managing weight and metabolism. As we age, our metabolism slows down, making it easier to gain weight. Regular exercise helps to burn calories and maintain a healthy weight. It also boosts energy levels, enhances mood, and reduces feelings of anxiety and depression.

Moreover, physical activity is essential for maintaining independence. Regular movement and exercise can help prevent falls by improving balance and coordination. This is particularly important for older adults, as falls can lead to serious injuries and complications.

Low-Impact Exercises and Routines

When it comes to exercise, it's important to choose activities that are safe and suitable for your fitness level. Low-impact exercises are gentle on the joints and reduce the risk of injury while still providing significant health benefits.

Walking is one of the best low-impact exercises. It's easy to incorporate into your daily routine and can be done almost anywhere. Aim for at least 30 minutes of brisk walking most days of the week. Walking helps improve cardiovascular health, strengthens muscles, and supports weight management.

Swimming and water aerobics are excellent options for those with joint pain or arthritis. The buoyancy of water reduces stress on the joints while providing resistance to build strength and improve cardiovascular fitness. Many community centers and gyms offer water exercise classes tailored for older adults.

Yoga is another great low-impact exercise that enhances flexibility, balance, and strength. There are many styles of yoga, and some are specifically designed for seniors. Chair yoga, for example, is a gentle form that can be done while seated or using a chair for support. Yoga also promotes relaxation and stress reduction.

Tai Chi is a traditional Chinese practice that involves slow, controlled movements and deep breathing. It's particularly beneficial for improving balance and coordination, which helps prevent falls. Tai Chi is also known for its calming effects and can help reduce stress and anxiety.

Strength training is important for maintaining muscle mass and bone density. Using light weights or resistance bands can help build strength without putting too much strain on the joints. Aim to include strength training exercises at least twice a week, focusing on all major muscle groups.

Stretching is essential for maintaining flexibility and preventing stiffness. Incorporate gentle stretches into your daily routine, focusing on the major muscle groups. Stretching helps improve range of motion and can alleviate muscle tension and soreness.

Tips for Enhancing Mobility

Maintaining mobility involves more than just regular exercise. There are several practical tips and strategies that can help you stay mobile and independent as you age.

First, it's important to listen to your body and recognize your limits. While regular exercise is beneficial, overexertion can lead to injury. Start slowly and gradually increase the intensity and duration of your activities. If you experience pain or discomfort, stop the activity and consult a healthcare provider.

Staying hydrated is crucial for maintaining mobility. Dehydration can lead to muscle cramps and weakness, which can affect your ability to move and exercise. Drink plenty of water throughout the day, especially before, during, and after physical activity.

Wearing appropriate footwear is also essential. Choose shoes that provide good support and cushioning to reduce the risk of falls and injuries. Avoid wearing slippers or shoes with slippery soles.

Incorporating physical activity into your daily routine can make it easier to stay active. Take the stairs instead of the elevator, park further away from the entrance, or take short walks during breaks. Even small amounts of physical activity can add up and make a significant difference.

Maintaining a healthy diet is important for supporting physical activity and overall health. Ensure you're getting enough protein to support muscle health, as well as vitamins and minerals like calcium and vitamin D for bone health. Eating a balanced diet rich in fruits, vegetables, whole grains, and lean proteins can provide the energy and nutrients needed for an active lifestyle.

Regular check-ups with your healthcare provider are important for monitoring your health and addressing any concerns that may affect your mobility. Discuss your exercise routine with your doctor, especially if you have any chronic conditions or are taking medications that may impact your ability to exercise safely.

Using assistive devices can help maintain independence and mobility. Canes, walkers, and other aids can provide support and stability, making it easier to move around safely. Consult a physical therapist or healthcare provider to determine the most suitable devices for your needs.

Creating a safe home environment can also enhance mobility and prevent falls. Remove tripping hazards like loose rugs and clutter, ensure good lighting, and install grab bars in areas like the bathroom. Keeping your living space organized and free of obstacles can reduce the risk of accidents.

Social support is another key factor in maintaining mobility. Exercising with friends or joining a group class can provide motivation and make physical activity more enjoyable. Social interactions also contribute to emotional well-being, which is closely linked to physical health.

Also, staying mentally active is important for overall mobility. Engaging in activities that stimulate the mind, such as puzzles, reading, or learning new skills, can improve cognitive function and coordination. A sharp mind supports better decision-making and reaction times, which are important for staying mobile and independent.

CHAPTER 4: BONE HEALTH AND OSTEOPOROSIS

Understanding Bone Density Loss

Bone density refers to the amount of bone mineral in bone tissue. As we age, bone density naturally decreases, which can lead to osteoporosis. This process starts earlier in women due to hormonal changes that occur during menopause. Estrogen, a hormone that helps maintain bone density, decreases significantly during menopause, accelerating bone loss.

The bones are living tissues that constantly break down and rebuild. In young adults, the rate of bone formation is faster than the rate of bone resorption, leading to an increase in bone mass. However, after the age of 30, the balance shifts, and bone resorption starts to outpace bone formation, resulting in a gradual loss of bone density.

Bone density loss can be measured using a bone density test, also known as a DEXA scan. This test helps diagnose osteoporosis and assess the risk of fractures. Regular bone density screenings are essential for women over 70 to monitor bone health and take timely action if needed.

Preventing and Managing Osteoporosis

Preventing and managing osteoporosis involves a combination of lifestyle changes, dietary adjustments, and medical treatments. Early intervention can significantly reduce the risk of fractures and improve quality of life.

Weight-bearing exercises are crucial for maintaining bone density. Activities such as walking, jogging, dancing, and resistance training help stimulate bone formation. These exercises put stress on the bones, which encourages the body to strengthen them. It's important to incorporate these activities into your routine several times a week.

In addition to weight-bearing exercises, balance and flexibility exercises, such as yoga and tai chi, can help prevent falls by improving stability and coordination. Falls are a major cause of fractures in older adults, so enhancing balance is key to reducing this risk.

Medications may be prescribed to help manage osteoporosis. Bisphosphonates are commonly used to slow down bone resorption, while medications like denosumab and teriparatide can help build bone mass. Hormone replacement therapy (HRT) can also be considered for postmenopausal women to maintain estrogen levels and support bone health. It's important to discuss the risks and benefits of these medications with a healthcare provider.

Lifestyle modifications can also play a significant role in preventing and managing osteoporosis. Avoiding smoking and limiting alcohol intake are crucial steps. Smoking has been shown to reduce bone density, and excessive alcohol consumption can interfere with the body's ability to absorb calcium, both of which increase the risk of osteoporosis.

Dietary and Lifestyle Recommendations

A balanced diet rich in essential nutrients is vital for maintaining strong bones. Calcium and vitamin D are particularly important for bone health. Calcium is the primary mineral found in bones, and vitamin D helps the body absorb calcium effectively.

Dairy products such as milk, yogurt, and cheese are excellent sources of calcium. For those who are lactose intolerant or prefer non-dairy options, leafy green vegetables like kale and broccoli, as well as fortified foods like almond milk and orange juice, can provide adequate calcium.

Vitamin D can be obtained from exposure to sunlight and from dietary sources. Fatty fish such as salmon and mackerel, as well as fortified foods like cereals and dairy products, are good sources of vitamin D. In some cases, supplements may be necessary to ensure adequate intake, especially in regions with limited sunlight.

Protein is another essential nutrient for bone health. It helps build and repair tissues, including bones. Incorporate lean proteins like poultry, fish, beans, and nuts into your diet to support overall bone strength.

Magnesium and potassium also play a role in bone health. Magnesium helps convert vitamin D into its active form, which aids in calcium absorption. Foods rich in magnesium include nuts, seeds, whole grains, and leafy green vegetables. Potassium helps neutralize acids that can remove calcium from the body, and it is found in foods like bananas, sweet potatoes, and spinach.

Maintaining a healthy weight is important for bone health. Being underweight can increase the risk of bone loss and fractures, while being overweight can put extra stress on the bones. A balanced diet and regular exercise can help achieve and maintain a healthy weight.

Staying hydrated is essential for overall health, including bone health. Water helps transport nutrients throughout the body and supports cellular functions. Aim to drink plenty of water throughout the day to stay hydrated.

In addition to dietary changes, it's important to create a safe living environment to prevent falls. Remove tripping hazards like loose rugs and ensure good lighting in all areas of your home. Installing grab bars in the bathroom and using non-slip mats can also reduce the risk of falls.

Regular check-ups with a healthcare provider are essential for monitoring bone health and managing osteoporosis. Discuss any concerns or symptoms with your doctor, and follow their recommendations for bone density screenings and medications if necessary.

PART III:

CARDIOVASCULAR AND CHRONIC HEALTH

CHAPTER 5:
CARDIOVASCULAR
HEALTH

Heart disease is a significant concern for women over 70. As we age, the risk of cardiovascular problems increases, making it crucial to understand the factors involved and adopt preventive measures. This chapter explores the prevalence of heart disease in older women, essential preventive measures and screenings, and the importance of a heart-healthy diet and lifestyle.

Heart Disease in Women Over 70

Heart disease remains a leading cause of death among older women. Several factors contribute to this increased risk, including age-related changes in the cardiovascular system, such as stiffening of the arteries and a decrease in the efficiency of the heart. These changes can lead to conditions like hypertension (high blood pressure), atherosclerosis (hardening of the arteries), and heart failure.

One common form of heart disease in older women is coronary artery disease (CAD), which occurs when the arteries that supply blood to the heart muscle become narrowed or blocked. This can result in chest pain (angina), shortness of breath, and, in severe cases, heart attacks.

Hypertension is another prevalent issue. High blood pressure can damage the arteries and lead to complications such as stroke, heart attack, and kidney damage. It's often called a "silent killer" because it usually doesn't cause symptoms until significant damage has occurred.

Atrial fibrillation (AFib) is an irregular heartbeat that becomes more common with age. It can lead to blood clots, stroke, and other heart-related complications. Women with AFib may experience palpitations, fatigue, or lightheadedness.

Preventive Measures and Screenings

Preventing heart disease involves a combination of lifestyle changes and regular medical screenings. Early detection and management of risk factors can significantly reduce the likelihood of developing serious cardiovascular problems.

Regular check-ups with a healthcare provider are essential for monitoring heart health. Blood pressure should be measured at every visit to detect hypertension early. Cholesterol levels should be checked periodically through blood tests. High levels of LDL (bad) cholesterol and low levels of HDL (good) cholesterol can increase the risk of heart disease.

Electrocardiograms (ECGs) and echocardiograms are non-invasive tests that can help diagnose heart conditions. An ECG measures the electrical activity of the heart and can detect arrhythmias, while an echocardiogram uses sound waves to create images of the heart, allowing doctors to assess its structure and function.

In addition to medical screenings, adopting heart-healthy habits is crucial. Smoking is a major risk factor for heart disease, and quitting smoking can significantly improve heart health. Even if you've smoked for many years, quitting can still reduce your risk.

Regular physical activity is another key component of heart health. Aim for at least 150 minutes of moderate-intensity aerobic exercise per week, such as brisk walking, swimming, or cycling. Exercise helps lower blood pressure, improve cholesterol levels, and maintain a healthy weight.

Managing stress is also important, as chronic stress can contribute to heart disease. Techniques such as mindfulness, meditation, and deep breathing exercises can help reduce stress levels. Engaging in hobbies, spending time with loved ones, and staying socially active can also promote emotional well-being.

Heart-Healthy Diet and Lifestyle

A heart-healthy diet plays a significant role in preventing and managing heart disease. Eating a balanced diet rich in fruits, vegetables, whole grains, lean proteins, and healthy fats can support cardiovascular health and reduce the risk of heart disease.

Fruits and vegetables are high in vitamins, minerals, and antioxidants that protect the heart. Aim to fill half your plate with a variety of colorful fruits and vegetables at each meal. Leafy greens, berries, and citrus fruits are particularly beneficial.

Whole grains, such as brown rice, oats, and whole wheat bread, provide essential nutrients and fiber that can help lower cholesterol levels and maintain a healthy weight. Replace refined grains with whole grains to improve heart health.

Lean proteins, such as poultry, fish, beans, and legumes, are important for maintaining muscle mass and overall health. Fish, especially fatty fish like salmon and mackerel, is rich in omega-3 fatty acids, which have been shown to reduce inflammation and lower the risk of heart disease.

Healthy fats, including those found in avocados, nuts, seeds, and olive oil, are beneficial for heart health. These fats can help reduce LDL cholesterol levels and improve HDL cholesterol levels. Avoid trans fats and limit saturated fats, which are found in processed foods and fatty cuts of meat, as they can increase the risk of heart disease.

Reducing sodium intake is essential for managing blood pressure. High sodium levels can lead to hypertension and other cardiovascular problems. Limit processed and packaged foods, which are often high in sodium, and opt for fresh, whole foods instead. Use herbs and spices to flavor your meals instead of salt.

Staying hydrated is also important for heart health. Drinking plenty of water helps maintain blood volume and supports overall bodily functions. Limit sugary drinks and alcohol, as excessive consumption can negatively impact heart health.

Maintaining a healthy weight is crucial for reducing the risk of heart disease. Excess weight, especially around the abdomen, can increase the risk of hypertension, diabetes, and high cholesterol. A balanced diet and regular physical activity can help achieve and maintain a healthy weight.

Sleep is another critical factor for heart health. Poor sleep quality and insufficient sleep can increase the risk of cardiovascular problems. Aim for 7-8 hours of quality sleep each night. Establish a regular sleep routine, create a comfortable sleep environment, and avoid caffeine and heavy meals before bedtime to improve sleep quality.

Incorporating these heart-healthy habits into your daily life can significantly reduce the risk of heart disease and improve overall well-being. Regular medical screenings, combined with a balanced diet, regular exercise, stress management, and adequate sleep, form the foundation of good cardiovascular health for women over 70. By taking proactive steps to care for your heart, you can enjoy a longer, healthier life with greater vitality and energy.

CHAPTER 6: MANAGING CHRONIC CONDITIONS

Diabetes: Prevention and Control

Diabetes is a chronic condition that affects how your body processes blood sugar (glucose). There are two main types: Type 1 diabetes, which is typically diagnosed in younger individuals and involves the body not producing insulin, and Type 2 diabetes, which is more common in older adults and involves the body becoming resistant to insulin or not producing enough of it.

Preventing Type 2 diabetes involves making lifestyle changes that can help maintain normal blood sugar levels. These include maintaining a healthy weight through diet and exercise. Eating a balanced diet rich in whole foods like fruits, vegetables, whole grains, and lean proteins can help regulate blood sugar levels. Limiting refined sugars and processed foods is also important.

Regular physical activity is essential for preventing and managing diabetes. Exercise helps the body use insulin more effectively and can lower blood sugar levels. Aim for at least 150 minutes of moderate-intensity aerobic activity each week, such as brisk walking, swimming, or cycling, combined with strength training exercises.

For those already diagnosed with diabetes, managing the condition involves regular monitoring of blood sugar levels, adhering to prescribed medications, and maintaining a healthy lifestyle. Blood sugar levels should be checked regularly to ensure they remain within the target range. Medications, such as metformin or insulin, may be prescribed to help control blood sugar levels.

Diet plays a crucial role in diabetes management. Eating smaller, balanced meals throughout the day can help keep blood sugar levels stable. Incorporating high-fiber foods, such as fruits, vegetables, and whole grains, can slow the absorption of sugar and prevent spikes in blood sugar levels.

Staying hydrated is also important, as dehydration can affect blood sugar levels. Drink plenty of water throughout the day and limit sugary drinks and alcohol.

Regular check-ups with a healthcare provider are essential for monitoring diabetes and preventing complications. These check-ups may include blood tests to monitor blood sugar levels, kidney function, and cholesterol levels. Foot exams are also important, as diabetes can lead to nerve damage and poor circulation, increasing the risk of foot problems.

Hypertension: Monitoring and Management

Hypertension, or high blood pressure, is a common condition in older adults that increases the risk of heart disease, stroke, and other health problems. Blood pressure is the force of blood pushing against the walls of the arteries. When this pressure is consistently too high, it can damage the arteries and lead to serious health issues.

Monitoring blood pressure regularly is key to managing hypertension. Blood pressure can be measured at home using a blood pressure monitor or at a healthcare provider's office. It's important to follow the doctor's recommendations on how often to check blood pressure and to keep a record of the readings.

Diet plays a significant role in managing hypertension. The DASH (Dietary Approaches to Stop Hypertension) diet is often recommended, which focuses on reducing sodium intake and eating a variety of nutrient-rich foods. Foods high in potassium, calcium, and magnesium can help control blood pressure. These include fruits, vegetables, whole grains, and low-fat dairy products.

Reducing sodium intake is crucial for lowering blood pressure. Limit processed and packaged foods, which are often high in sodium, and opt for fresh, whole foods instead. Use herbs and spices to flavor meals instead of salt.

Regular physical activity helps lower blood pressure by strengthening the heart and improving circulation. Aim for at least 150 minutes of moderate-intensity aerobic exercise each week. Activities like walking, swimming, and cycling are beneficial.

Weight management is also important, as being overweight can increase the risk of hypertension. A balanced diet and regular exercise can help achieve and maintain a healthy weight.

Limiting alcohol consumption and quitting smoking are critical steps in managing hypertension. Alcohol can raise blood pressure, and smoking damages the arteries, increasing the risk of heart disease.

Medications may be prescribed to help control blood pressure. These can include diuretics, ACE inhibitors, beta-blockers, and calcium channel blockers. It's important to take medications as prescribed and to discuss any side effects with a healthcare provider.

Stress management techniques, such as mindfulness, meditation, and deep breathing exercises, can help reduce stress levels, which can positively impact blood pressure. Engaging in hobbies and spending time with loved ones can also promote relaxation and emotional well-being.

Arthritis: Types, Pain Management, and Physical Therapy

Arthritis is a condition that causes inflammation and pain in the joints. It is common among older adults, with osteoarthritis and rheumatoid arthritis being the most prevalent types. Osteoarthritis is caused by wear and tear on the joints, while rheumatoid arthritis is an autoimmune condition where the immune system attacks the joints.

Managing arthritis involves a combination of lifestyle changes, pain management strategies, and physical therapy. Staying active is crucial for maintaining joint function and reducing stiffness. Low-impact exercises, such as walking, swimming, and yoga, can help improve flexibility and strength without putting too much strain on the joints.

Weight management is important for reducing stress on the joints. Excess weight can exacerbate arthritis symptoms, so maintaining a healthy weight through a balanced diet and regular exercise is beneficial.

Pain management strategies can include over-the-counter medications, such as acetaminophen or nonsteroidal anti-inflammatory drugs (NSAIDs). In some cases, stronger prescription medications or corticosteroid injections may be necessary to manage severe pain and inflammation.

Physical therapy can be highly effective in managing arthritis symptoms. A physical therapist can develop a personalized exercise program to improve joint function, increase strength, and reduce pain. Techniques such as heat and cold therapy, ultrasound, and electrical stimulation may also be used to alleviate symptoms.

Assistive devices, such as braces, splints, or canes, can provide support and reduce strain on the joints. It's important to use these devices as recommended by a healthcare provider or physical therapist.

Diet can also play a role in managing arthritis. Anti-inflammatory foods, such as fatty fish, nuts, seeds, fruits, and vegetables, can help reduce inflammation in the body. Omega-3 fatty acids, found in fish and flaxseeds, are particularly beneficial.

Regular check-ups with a healthcare provider are essential for monitoring arthritis and adjusting treatment plans as needed. Discuss any changes in symptoms or new concerns with the doctor to ensure appropriate management of the condition.

PART IV:

COGNITIVE AND MENTAL HEALTH

CHAPTER 7: COGNITIVE HEALTH AND DEMENTIA

Understanding Cognitive Decline

As we grow older, some degree of cognitive decline is a normal part of aging. This can include slower processing speeds, occasional memory lapses, and reduced multitasking ability. However, these changes do not necessarily indicate dementia. It's essential to distinguish between normal age-related changes and more serious conditions.

Cognitive decline can be influenced by various factors, including genetics, lifestyle, and overall health. Conditions such as hypertension, diabetes, and cardiovascular disease can contribute to cognitive impairment. Additionally, lifestyle choices such as diet, physical activity, and mental engagement play significant roles in cognitive health.

Research shows that the brain can continue to form new connections throughout life, a concept known as neuroplasticity. Engaging in activities that challenge the brain, such as learning new skills, solving puzzles, or engaging in social activities, can help maintain cognitive function.

Early Signs of Dementia

Dementia is a general term for a decline in cognitive function severe enough to interfere with daily life. Alzheimer's disease is the most common form of dementia, but there are other types, including vascular dementia, Lewy body dementia, and frontotemporal dementia.

Recognizing the early signs of dementia is crucial for early intervention and management. Common early symptoms include:

1. **Memory Loss:** Frequently forgetting recent events, names, or places. While occasional forgetfulness is normal, persistent memory loss that disrupts daily life may be a sign of dementia.

2. **Difficulty Performing Familiar Tasks:** Struggling to complete everyday tasks, such as cooking, managing finances, or driving, which were previously done with ease.

3. **Problems with Language:** Difficulty finding the right words, following conversations, or understanding written and spoken language.

4. **Disorientation:** Becoming confused about time or place, such as getting lost in familiar surroundings or forgetting the date.

5. **Poor Judgment:** Making uncharacteristic decisions or exhibiting poor judgment in personal and financial matters.

6. **Changes in Mood and Behavior:** Experiencing mood swings, anxiety, depression, or sudden changes in personality. This can include

becoming withdrawn, irritable, or apathetic.

7. **Loss of Initiative:** Losing interest in activities and hobbies that were once enjoyable, and showing a lack of motivation.

If you or a loved one experiences these symptoms, it is important to seek medical advice. Early diagnosis can help manage the symptoms and improve quality of life.

Strategies for Maintaining Cognitive Function

Maintaining cognitive function involves a combination of lifestyle changes, mental exercises, and social engagement. Here are some strategies to support cognitive health:

1. **Regular Physical Activity:** Exercise has been shown to improve cognitive function and reduce the risk of dementia. Activities such as walking, swimming, and yoga promote blood

flow to the brain and support overall brain health.

2. **Healthy Diet:** A balanced diet rich in fruits, vegetables, whole grains, lean proteins, and healthy fats can support cognitive function. The Mediterranean diet, which includes plenty of fish, nuts, and olive oil, has been associated with a lower risk of cognitive decline.

3. **Mental Stimulation:** Engage in activities that challenge your brain, such as puzzles, reading, playing musical instruments, or learning a new language. These activities can help maintain and improve cognitive function.

4. **Social Interaction:** Staying socially active is important for cognitive health. Regular interactions with friends, family, and community groups can provide emotional support and mental stimulation. Volunteering, joining clubs, or participating in group

activities can help maintain social connections.

5. **Adequate Sleep:** Quality sleep is essential for brain health. Aim for 7-8 hours of sleep each night. Establish a regular sleep routine, create a comfortable sleep environment, and avoid caffeine and electronic devices before bedtime to improve sleep quality.

6. **Stress Management:** Chronic stress can negatively impact cognitive function. Techniques such as mindfulness, meditation, and deep breathing exercises can help manage stress. Engaging in hobbies and spending time in nature can also promote relaxation and reduce stress levels.

7. **Regular Check-Ups:** Regular medical check-ups can help monitor cognitive health and identify any potential issues early. Discuss any concerns with your healthcare

provider and follow their recommendations for screenings and tests.

8. **Manage Chronic Conditions:** Managing chronic conditions such as hypertension, diabetes, and cardiovascular disease is important for cognitive health. Follow your healthcare provider's advice on medications, diet, and lifestyle changes to keep these conditions under control.

9. **Stay Mentally Active:** Continuously seek opportunities to learn and challenge your brain. Take up new hobbies, enroll in courses, or participate in lifelong learning programs. Keeping your brain active and engaged can help maintain cognitive function.

10. **Avoid Smoking and Limit Alcohol:** Smoking and excessive alcohol consumption can increase the risk of cognitive decline. Quitting

smoking and limiting alcohol intake can support overall brain health.

By incorporating these strategies into your daily routine, you can support cognitive health and reduce the risk of dementia. Maintaining a healthy lifestyle, staying mentally and socially active, and managing stress are all key components of preserving cognitive function as you age.

CHAPTER 8: MENTAL HEALTH AND EMOTIONAL WELL-BEING

Mental health and emotional well-being are critical components of overall health, particularly for older adults. As we age, we may encounter various emotional challenges and changes that can impact our mental health. It's essential to recognize these changes, understand the signs of mental health issues like depression and anxiety, and adopt effective coping mechanisms and support systems. Additionally, maintaining social connections plays a significant role in promoting emotional well-being.

Recognizing Depression and Anxiety

Depression and anxiety are common mental health issues that can affect anyone, including older adults. These conditions may be triggered by various factors such as health problems, loss of loved ones, or significant life changes. Recognizing the signs of depression and anxiety is the first step towards seeking help and managing these conditions effectively.

Depression in older adults may present differently than in younger individuals. Common signs of depression include persistent sadness, feelings of hopelessness or helplessness, loss of interest in activities once enjoyed, changes in appetite or weight, difficulty sleeping or sleeping too much, and fatigue. Older adults may also experience physical symptoms such as aches and pains that do not have a clear medical cause.

Anxiety can manifest as excessive worry, restlessness, irritability, difficulty concentrating, and physical symptoms like muscle tension, headaches, and an increased heart rate. Anxiety in older adults can be related to health concerns, financial worries, or fear of losing independence.

It's important to note that these symptoms can vary in intensity and may overlap with other medical conditions. Therefore, seeking a professional evaluation from a healthcare provider is crucial for an accurate diagnosis and appropriate treatment.

Coping Mechanisms and Support Systems

Developing effective coping mechanisms and building a strong support system are essential for managing depression and anxiety. These strategies can help improve mental health and enhance emotional well-being.

One of the most effective coping mechanisms is staying physically active. Regular exercise, such as walking, swimming, or yoga, can boost mood, reduce stress, and improve overall mental health. Physical activity releases endorphins, which are natural mood lifters, and can also help alleviate symptoms of anxiety and depression.

Engaging in hobbies and activities that bring joy and fulfillment can also have a positive impact on mental health. Whether it's gardening, painting, reading, or playing a musical instrument, finding activities that you enjoy can provide a sense of purpose and satisfaction.

Mindfulness and relaxation techniques, such as meditation, deep breathing exercises, and progressive muscle relaxation, can help manage stress and anxiety. Practicing mindfulness can improve focus, reduce negative thoughts, and promote a sense of calm and well-being.

Talking to someone about your feelings is another effective way to cope with depression and anxiety. This could be a trusted friend, family member, or mental health professional. Therapy or counseling can provide a safe space to explore your emotions, develop coping strategies, and receive support.

Support groups can also be beneficial for mental health. Joining a support group with others who are experiencing similar challenges can provide a sense of community and understanding. These groups can offer emotional support, practical advice, and a platform to share experiences.

Maintaining a healthy lifestyle is crucial for mental health. Eating a balanced diet rich in fruits, vegetables, whole grains, lean proteins, and healthy fats can support brain health and improve mood. Avoiding excessive caffeine and alcohol, which can exacerbate anxiety and depression, is also important.

Getting enough sleep is vital for emotional well-being. Poor sleep can worsen symptoms of depression and anxiety, so it's important to establish a regular sleep routine. Creating a comfortable sleep environment, avoiding screens before bedtime, and practicing relaxation techniques can help improve sleep quality.

The Importance of Social Connections

Social connections play a vital role in promoting mental health and emotional well-being. Staying socially active and maintaining relationships with family, friends, and the community can provide emotional support, reduce feelings of loneliness, and enhance overall happiness.

Engaging in social activities, such as joining clubs, volunteering, or participating in community events, can help build and maintain social connections. These activities provide opportunities to meet new people, develop friendships, and feel a sense of belonging.

Maintaining regular contact with family and friends is essential. This can be through phone calls, video chats, or in-person visits. Social interactions can provide emotional support, reduce stress, and improve mood.

Pets can also be a source of companionship and emotional support. Many older adults find joy and comfort in caring for pets, which can provide a sense of purpose and reduce feelings of loneliness.

It's important to recognize that building and maintaining social connections can take effort, especially if mobility or health issues are a concern. However, the benefits of staying socially active are significant and can greatly enhance emotional well-being.

In addition to personal efforts, community resources and services can support social connections. Many communities offer programs and activities specifically for older adults, such as senior centers, recreational classes, and social clubs. These programs can provide opportunities for social interaction and engagement.

For those who may have difficulty leaving their homes, online communities and virtual social groups can be valuable resources. Technology can help bridge the gap and keep people connected, even when physical distance is a barrier.

CHAPTER 9: NUTRITIONAL NEEDS FOR WOMEN OVER 70

Key Nutrients for Aging Gracefully

As we age, our bodies require different nutrients to maintain optimal function and health. Some key nutrients become particularly important for women over 70:

Calcium and Vitamin D: These nutrients are essential for maintaining bone health. Calcium supports bone density, while vitamin D helps the body absorb calcium. Sources of calcium include dairy products, leafy green vegetables, and fortified foods. Vitamin D can be obtained from sunlight, fatty fish, and fortified foods.

Protein: Protein is crucial for preserving muscle mass and strength, which tend to decline with age. It also supports the immune system and repairs body tissues.

Good sources of protein include lean meats, poultry, fish, eggs, beans, legumes, and dairy products.

Fiber: Fiber aids in digestion, helps prevent constipation, and can reduce the risk of heart disease. Whole grains, fruits, vegetables, nuts, and seeds are excellent sources of dietary fiber.

Omega-3 Fatty Acids: These healthy fats have anti-inflammatory properties and support heart and brain health. They are found in fatty fish like salmon, mackerel, and sardines, as well as in flaxseeds, chia seeds, and walnuts.

B Vitamins: B vitamins, particularly B12, are important for energy production, brain function, and the formation of red blood cells. As people age, the ability to absorb B12 decreases. Sources include meat, fish, dairy products, and fortified cereals.

Antioxidants: Vitamins C and E, as well as other antioxidants, protect cells from damage caused by free radicals. These can be found in a variety of fruits and vegetables, such as berries, citrus fruits, nuts, and seeds.

Magnesium: This mineral supports muscle and nerve function, helps regulate blood pressure, and contributes to bone health. Foods rich in magnesium include nuts, seeds, whole grains, and leafy green vegetables.

Potassium: Potassium helps maintain normal blood pressure and supports muscle and nerve function. It is found in bananas, oranges, potatoes, and spinach.

Water: Hydration is crucial for overall health. As people age, they may not feel thirsty as often, but it's important to drink enough water to prevent dehydration. Aim for at least 8 glasses of water a day.

Dietary Recommendations and Meal Plans

Creating a balanced diet that includes these key nutrients can help women over 70 maintain their health and vitality. Here are some dietary recommendations and sample meal plans to guide healthy eating:

- **Breakfast:** Start the day with a nutrient-rich breakfast. Options include oatmeal topped with berries and nuts, a vegetable omelet with whole-grain toast, or Greek yogurt with fruit and a sprinkle of flaxseeds.

- **Lunch:** Focus on lean proteins and plenty of vegetables. A salad with mixed greens, grilled chicken, avocado, and a light vinaigrette is a great choice. Another option is a quinoa bowl with roasted vegetables, chickpeas, and a tahini dressing.

- **Dinner:** Include a variety of foods to ensure a balanced intake of nutrients.

Consider baked salmon with a side of steamed broccoli and brown rice, or a stir-fry with tofu, colorful vegetables, and whole-grain noodles.

- **Snacks:** Choose healthy snacks that provide energy and nutrients. Options include a handful of almonds, carrot sticks with hummus, or a piece of fruit.

- **Hydration:** Ensure adequate fluid intake by drinking water throughout the day. Herbal teas and water-rich fruits and vegetables like cucumbers and watermelon can also help with hydration.

When planning meals, it's important to incorporate a variety of foods to meet nutritional needs. A balanced plate should include proteins, healthy fats, fiber-rich carbohydrates, and plenty of fruits and vegetables.

Supplements and Their Role

While a well-balanced diet is the best way to obtain necessary nutrients, supplements can play a role in ensuring adequate intake, especially when dietary sources are insufficient. It's important to use supplements judiciously and under the guidance of a healthcare provider.

Calcium and Vitamin D Supplements: For those who have difficulty getting enough calcium and vitamin D from food and sunlight, supplements can help maintain bone health. It's essential to choose the right dosage to avoid potential side effects.

Multivitamins: A daily multivitamin can help fill nutritional gaps and ensure adequate intake of essential vitamins and minerals. Look for formulations specifically designed for older adults, which typically contain higher levels of certain nutrients like B12 and vitamin D.

Omega-3 Supplements: Fish oil supplements can provide omega-3 fatty acids if dietary intake is low. These supplements support heart and brain health and have anti-inflammatory benefits.

B12 Supplements: Given the decreased ability to absorb B12 with age, a supplement can help maintain adequate levels. B12 is available in various forms, including tablets, sublingual (under the tongue) drops, and injections.

Magnesium Supplements: If dietary intake is insufficient, a magnesium supplement can support muscle and nerve function, as well as bone health.

Fiber Supplements: For those who have difficulty getting enough fiber from food, supplements like psyllium husk can help maintain digestive health and regularity.

Probiotics: These supplements can support gut health and improve digestion. Probiotics are beneficial bacteria that can be found in fermented foods like yogurt and kefir, as well as in supplement form.

It's important to remember that supplements are not a substitute for a healthy diet. They should be used to complement dietary intake and address specific deficiencies. Before starting any supplement regimen, consult with a healthcare provider to ensure it's safe and appropriate for your individual needs.

By focusing on a balanced diet rich in essential nutrients, women over 70 can support their overall health and well-being. Proper nutrition plays a vital role in maintaining energy levels, cognitive function, bone health, and immune system strength. Combined with regular physical activity, adequate hydration, and appropriate supplementation, a nutrient-rich diet can help promote a long and healthy life.

CHAPTER 10: CANCER SCREENING AND PREVENTION

Common Cancers in Women Over 70

Several types of cancer are more prevalent in older women. Understanding these common cancers can help in recognizing symptoms early and seeking timely medical advice.

Breast cancer is one of the most common cancers among women. The risk increases with age, making regular mammograms essential for early detection. Symptoms can include a lump in the breast, changes in breast shape or size, dimpling of the skin, or nipple discharge. Regular self-examinations and clinical breast exams can also help detect abnormalities early.

Colorectal cancer affects the colon or rectum and is more common in older adults.

Symptoms can include changes in bowel habits, blood in the stool, abdominal pain, and unexplained weight loss. Regular screenings, such as colonoscopies, can detect precancerous polyps and early-stage colorectal cancer, improving the chances of successful treatment.

Lung cancer is another significant concern, especially for women with a history of smoking. Symptoms include a persistent cough, chest pain, shortness of breath, and coughing up blood. Low-dose CT scans are recommended for those at high risk, particularly former or current smokers.

Ovarian cancer often goes undetected until it has spread within the pelvis and abdomen. Symptoms can be vague and include bloating, pelvic pain, and changes in bowel habits. Regular pelvic exams and awareness of family history can aid in early detection.

Skin cancer, including melanoma and non-melanoma types, is common among older adults. Changes in the skin, such as new growths, sores that don't heal, or changes in existing moles, should be examined by a healthcare provider. Regular skin checks and protection from UV radiation are crucial preventive measures.

Recommended Screenings and Tests

Regular screenings are vital for early detection and treatment of cancer. Here are some recommended screenings and tests for women over 70:

Mammograms are essential for detecting breast cancer. Women over 70 should have mammograms every one to two years, depending on their risk factors and overall health. Discuss with your healthcare provider to determine the appropriate screening schedule.

Colonoscopy is the gold standard for colorectal cancer screening. It is recommended every ten years for those with average risk, but more frequent screenings may be needed for those with higher risk factors. Alternatives include stool tests and flexible sigmoidoscopy, but colonoscopy remains the most comprehensive.

Low-dose CT scans are recommended for lung cancer screening in high-risk individuals, particularly those with a significant smoking history. This annual screening can detect early-stage lung cancer, improving treatment outcomes.

Pelvic exams and transvaginal ultrasounds can help detect ovarian cancer. While there is no standard screening test for ovarian cancer, these exams can identify abnormalities that warrant further investigation. Women with a family history of ovarian or breast cancer should discuss genetic testing with their healthcare provider.

Pap smears and HPV tests are essential for detecting cervical cancer. While guidelines typically recommend stopping these screenings after age 65, women with a history of cervical cancer or pre-cancer should continue screenings as advised by their healthcare provider.

Skin checks should be performed regularly by a dermatologist, especially for those with a history of skin cancer or significant sun exposure. Self-examinations should also be done monthly to identify any new or changing skin lesions.

Blood tests and imaging studies, such as CT scans and MRIs, may be used to monitor for cancer recurrence in those with a history of cancer. Regular follow-ups with a healthcare provider are crucial for managing ongoing health and detecting any new issues early.

Lifestyle Choices for Cancer Prevention

Adopting a healthy lifestyle can significantly reduce the risk of developing cancer. Here are some lifestyle choices that can help prevent cancer:

Avoiding tobacco is one of the most important steps in cancer prevention. Smoking and using tobacco products are linked to various cancers, including lung, throat, mouth, and bladder cancer. Quitting smoking at any age can reduce the risk of developing cancer and improve overall health.

Eating a balanced diet rich in fruits, vegetables, whole grains, and lean proteins can provide essential nutrients that support overall health and reduce cancer risk. Limiting red meat and processed meats, which have been linked to an increased risk of colorectal cancer, is also beneficial.

Maintaining a healthy weight is crucial for cancer prevention. Obesity is associated with an increased risk of several cancers, including breast, colorectal, and endometrial cancer. Regular physical activity and a balanced diet can help achieve and maintain a healthy weight.

Regular physical activity is essential for overall health and can reduce the risk of several types of cancer. Aim for at least 150 minutes of moderate-intensity exercise or 75 minutes of vigorous-intensity exercise each week. Activities such as walking, swimming, cycling, and yoga can help keep the body healthy and reduce cancer risk.

Limiting alcohol consumption can also reduce the risk of developing cancer. Alcohol is linked to an increased risk of several cancers, including breast, liver, and colorectal cancer. Women should limit alcohol intake to one drink per day or less.

Protecting your skin from excessive sun exposure can prevent skin cancer. Use sunscreen with an SPF of 30 or higher, wear protective clothing, and avoid tanning beds. Regularly check your skin for any changes and seek medical advice for any suspicious lesions.

Getting vaccinated can prevent certain cancers. The HPV vaccine protects against the human papillomavirus, which can cause cervical, anal, and other cancers. The hepatitis B vaccine can reduce the risk of liver cancer. Discuss vaccination options with your healthcare provider.

Regular screenings and check-ups are essential for early detection and prevention of cancer. Follow the recommended screening guidelines for your age and risk factors. Early detection can significantly improve treatment outcomes and survival rates.

Managing stress and prioritizing mental health can also support overall well-being and potentially reduce cancer risk. Chronic stress can weaken the immune system and make the body more susceptible to illness. Practices such as mindfulness, meditation, and deep breathing exercises can help manage stress.

Avoiding exposure to harmful substances, such as asbestos and certain chemicals, can also reduce the risk of cancer. Follow safety guidelines and use protective equipment if you work in environments with potential carcinogens.

Staying informed and educated about cancer risk factors and prevention strategies is crucial. Regularly consult with healthcare providers, stay updated on the latest research, and take proactive steps to protect your health.

CHAPTER 11: REGULAR HEALTH CHECK-UPS

Importance of Routine Check-Ups

Routine check-ups play a vital role in preventive healthcare. They provide an opportunity to catch health issues early before they develop into more serious conditions. Early detection often leads to more effective treatment and better outcomes. For older adults, regular check-ups are especially important due to the increased risk of chronic diseases such as hypertension, diabetes, heart disease, and cancer.

Preventive screenings conducted during routine check-ups can identify risk factors and detect diseases at an early stage. For example, blood pressure measurements can identify hypertension, cholesterol tests can reveal cardiovascular risks, and blood glucose tests can detect diabetes. Screenings for certain types of cancer, such as mammograms and colonoscopies, can also be part of routine check-ups.

Regular check-ups are also important for managing existing health conditions. For those with chronic illnesses, these appointments allow for monitoring disease progression, adjusting medications, and implementing lifestyle changes to manage symptoms and improve quality of life. They also provide a platform for discussing any new symptoms or concerns with your healthcare provider.

In addition to detecting and managing health conditions, routine check-ups are essential for receiving vaccinations and immunizations. Older adults may need vaccines such as the flu shot, pneumococcal vaccine, and shingles vaccine to protect against infections. Staying up-to-date with vaccinations can prevent serious illnesses and complications.

Mental health is another critical aspect of overall well-being that can be addressed during routine check-ups. Regular appointments provide an opportunity to discuss any mental health concerns, such as anxiety or depression, and receive appropriate referrals for counseling or therapy if needed.

What to Expect During Health Appointments

Knowing what to expect during health appointments can help you prepare and make the most of your time with your healthcare provider. Here are some key components of a typical check-up:

- **Medical History Review:** Your healthcare provider will review your medical history, including any chronic conditions, past surgeries, medications, allergies, and family medical history. This information helps the provider understand your overall health and identify any potential risk factors.

- **Physical Examination:** A thorough physical exam is conducted to assess your general health. This may include measuring your height, weight, and blood pressure, as well as examining your heart, lungs, abdomen, skin, and extremities. Your provider may also check your reflexes, vision, and hearing.

- **Screenings and Tests:** Based on your age, medical history, and risk factors, your healthcare provider may recommend various screenings and tests. These can include blood tests to check cholesterol and glucose levels, bone density tests to assess the risk of osteoporosis, and cancer screenings such as mammograms, Pap smears, or colonoscopies.

- **Discussion of Symptoms:** It's important to discuss any new or ongoing symptoms you may be experiencing. Be open and honest about how you feel, as this information is crucial for accurate diagnosis and treatment. Common symptoms to report include changes in weight, sleep patterns, appetite, energy levels, and mood.

- **Medication Review:** Your healthcare provider will review your current medications, including prescriptions, over-the-counter drugs, and supplements. This ensures that you are taking the correct dosages and helps identify any potential interactions or side effects. Be sure to bring a list of all medications and supplements you are currently taking.

- **Vaccinations:** Depending on your age and medical history, your provider may recommend certain vaccinations to protect against infections. Common vaccines for older adults include the flu shot, pneumococcal vaccine, shingles vaccine, and tetanus booster.

- **Health Counseling:** During the appointment, your healthcare provider may offer advice on lifestyle changes to improve your health. This can include recommendations for a balanced diet, regular exercise, smoking cessation, and alcohol moderation. They may also provide guidance on managing stress and improving mental health.

- **Referrals and Follow-Up:** If any issues are identified during the check-up, your provider may refer you to a specialist for further evaluation and treatment. They will also schedule follow-up appointments to monitor your progress and ensure that any health concerns are being addressed effectively.

Building a Relationship with Your Healthcare Provider

Building a strong relationship with your healthcare provider is essential for effective healthcare. A good provider-patient relationship is based on trust, communication, and mutual respect. Here are some tips for fostering a positive relationship with your healthcare provider:

Be Open and Honest: Share all relevant information about your health, including symptoms, lifestyle habits, and any concerns you may have. Honesty is crucial for accurate diagnosis and effective treatment. Don't hesitate to ask questions if you don't understand something or need more information.

Prepare for Appointments: Write down any questions or concerns you have before your appointment. Bring a list of all medications and supplements you are taking. Being prepared can help ensure that you cover all important topics during the visit.

Communicate Clearly: Clearly describe your symptoms, how long they have been present, and how they affect your daily life.

Provide as much detail as possible to help your provider understand your condition.

Follow Recommendations: Adhere to the treatment plan and follow the advice provided by your healthcare provider. If you have any difficulties with the prescribed treatment, discuss them with your provider to find alternative solutions.

Stay Informed: Educate yourself about your health conditions and treatment options. Reliable sources of information can help you make informed decisions about your care. Your healthcare provider can recommend trustworthy resources.

Build Trust: Trust is a key component of a strong provider-patient relationship. Trust your provider's expertise and judgment, and communicate openly about any concerns or preferences you have regarding your care.

Schedule Regular Appointments: Regular check-ups are essential for maintaining health. Even if you feel well, routine visits allow your provider to monitor your health and catch any potential issues early. Don't wait until you are sick to see your healthcare provider.

Seek a Second Opinion if Needed: If you have concerns about your diagnosis or treatment plan, it's okay to seek a second opinion. Another healthcare provider can offer a fresh perspective and additional insights.

Respect Your Provider's Time: Be punctual for your appointments and understand that your provider may have other patients to see. Respecting their time helps ensure that appointments run smoothly and efficiently.

Express Gratitude: A simple thank you can go a long way in building a positive relationship. Expressing gratitude for your provider's care and attention fosters a respectful and supportive environment.

By following these tips, you can build a strong, trusting relationship with your healthcare provider. This partnership is essential for effective health management and ensures that you receive the best possible care. Regular health check-ups, open communication, and mutual respect are the foundations of a successful provider-patient relationship. Taking an active role in your healthcare and working closely with your provider will help you maintain optimal health and well-being as you age.

CONCLUSION: EMBRACING YOUR GOLDEN YEARS

Recap of Key Points

Throughout this book, we have explored various aspects of health and wellness for women over 70. Here are some key takeaways:

Maintaining Mobility and Physical Activity: Regular exercise, such as walking, swimming, and yoga, is crucial for maintaining mobility, strength, and overall health. Low-impact exercises can help prevent injuries while keeping you active and engaged.

Bone Health and Osteoporosis: Ensuring adequate intake of calcium and vitamin D, along with weight-bearing exercises, can help maintain bone density and prevent osteoporosis. Regular bone density screenings are also important.

Cardiovascular Health: Monitoring blood pressure and cholesterol levels, maintaining a heart-healthy diet, and engaging in regular physical activity are essential for cardiovascular health. Regular check-ups and screenings can detect issues early.

Managing Chronic Conditions: Managing diabetes, hypertension, and arthritis involves a combination of medication, lifestyle changes, and regular monitoring. A balanced diet, regular exercise, and adherence to treatment plans are key components.

Cognitive Health and Dementia: Engaging in mentally stimulating activities, staying socially active, and managing chronic conditions can help maintain cognitive function. Early detection of dementia symptoms is crucial for effective management.

Mental Health and Emotional Well-being: Recognizing and addressing symptoms of depression and anxiety, developing coping mechanisms, and building strong support systems are essential for emotional well-being. Social connections play a significant role in mental health.

Nutritional Needs and Dietary Guidance: A balanced diet rich in essential nutrients, including protein, fiber, vitamins, and minerals, is vital for overall health. Supplements can help fill nutritional gaps when necessary.

Cancer Screening and Prevention: Regular screenings for breast, colorectal, lung, and skin cancers are important for early detection and treatment. Adopting a healthy lifestyle can reduce the risk of cancer.

Regular Health Check-Ups: Routine check-ups and screenings are essential for monitoring health and detecting potential issues early. Building a strong relationship with your healthcare provider is crucial for effective health management.

Staying Motivated and Positive

Maintaining motivation and a positive outlook is essential for enjoying your golden years. Here are some strategies to help you stay motivated and positive:

- **Set Realistic Goals:** Setting achievable goals gives you a sense of purpose and direction. Whether it's starting a new hobby, improving your fitness level, or learning something new, setting and working towards goals can be very fulfilling.

- **Celebrate Small Wins:** Acknowledge and celebrate your accomplishments, no matter how small. Recognizing your progress helps boost confidence and motivation.

- **Stay Connected:** Maintain relationships with family and friends, and seek out new social opportunities. Social interactions provide emotional support and contribute to a positive mindset.

- **Practice Gratitude:** Take time each day to reflect on the things you are grateful for. Keeping a gratitude journal can help you focus on the positive aspects of your life.

- **Stay Active:** Physical activity has numerous benefits for both physical and mental health. Find activities you enjoy and make them a regular part of your routine.

- **Engage in Hobbies:** Pursue hobbies and activities that bring you joy and satisfaction. Engaging in creative and enjoyable pursuits can enhance your sense of well-being.

- **Seek Support:** If you're feeling down or overwhelmed, don't hesitate to seek support from friends, family, or mental health professionals. Talking about your feelings can provide relief and help you find solutions.

- **Stay Informed:** Educate yourself about health and wellness topics. Staying informed empowers you to make informed decisions about your health and well-being.

- **Practice Self-Compassion:** Be kind to yourself and recognize that it's okay to have bad days. Practicing self-compassion involves treating yourself with the same kindness and understanding that you would offer to a friend.

- **Embrace Change:** Aging brings changes, and embracing these changes with a positive attitude can make the transition smoother. Focus on the opportunities and experiences that come with each stage of life.

BONUS CHAPTER

Sample Meal Plans and Recipes

Maintaining a healthy and balanced diet is crucial for overall well-being, especially as we age. This section provides nutritious and easy-to-prepare recipes along with meal plans tailored to different dietary needs. Each recipe includes a brief description of its health benefits, detailed nutritional information, and step-by-step preparation instructions.

Nutritious and Easy-to-Prepare Recipes

Quinoa and Vegetable Stir-Fry

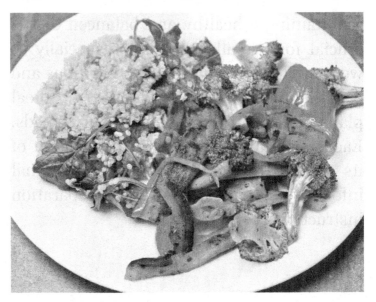

This recipe is rich in fiber, protein, and antioxidants. Quinoa is a complete protein, meaning it contains all nine essential amino acids. The colorful vegetables provide vitamins, minerals, and phytonutrients that support overall health and help reduce inflammation.

Nutritional Information (per serving):

- Calories: 320
- Protein: 12g
- Carbohydrates: 52g
- Dietary Fiber: 8g
- Sugars: 6g
- Fat: 8g
- Saturated Fat: 1g
- Sodium: 300mg

Ingredients:

- 1 cup quinoa
- 2 cups vegetable broth or water
- 1 tablespoon olive oil
- 1 small onion, chopped
- 2 cloves garlic, minced
- 1 red bell pepper, sliced
- 1 yellow bell pepper, sliced
- 1 zucchini, sliced
- 1 cup broccoli florets
- 2 tablespoons soy sauce (low sodium)
- 1 tablespoon sesame seeds
- Fresh cilantro for garnish

Preparation Instructions:

1. Rinse quinoa under cold water. In a medium saucepan, bring vegetable broth or water to a boil. Add quinoa, reduce heat to low, cover, and simmer for 15 minutes or until the liquid is absorbed. Fluff with a fork and set aside.

2. In a large skillet, heat olive oil over medium heat. Add onion and garlic, sauté for 2-3 minutes until fragrant.

3. Add red and yellow bell peppers, zucchini, and broccoli to the skillet. Cook for 5-7 minutes until vegetables are tender but still crisp.

4. Stir in cooked quinoa and soy sauce. Toss to combine and heat through.

5. Sprinkle with sesame seeds and garnish with fresh cilantro before serving.

Baked Salmon with Lemon and Dill

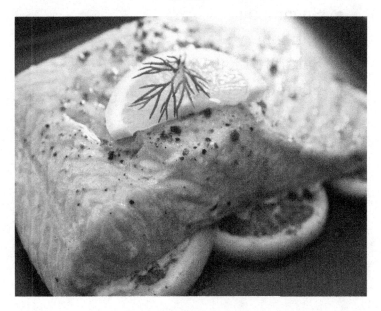

Salmon is an excellent source of omega-3 fatty acids, which support heart and brain health. This dish is also high in protein and provides essential vitamins and minerals such as vitamin D, B vitamins, and selenium.

Nutritional Information (per serving):
- Calories: 350
- Protein: 30g

- Carbohydrates: 2g
- Dietary Fiber: 1g
- Sugars: 0g
- Fat: 24g
- Saturated Fat: 4g
- Sodium: 180mg

Ingredients:
- 4 salmon fillets (about 6 oz each)
- 2 tablespoons olive oil
- 1 lemon, thinly sliced
- 2 tablespoons fresh dill, chopped
- Salt and pepper to taste
- 1 lemon, cut into wedges (for serving)

Preparation Instructions:
1. Preheat the oven to 375°F (190°C). Line a baking sheet with parchment paper.
2. Place salmon fillets on the prepared baking sheet. Drizzle with olive oil and season with salt and pepper.
3. Arrange lemon slices on top of the salmon fillets and sprinkle with fresh dill.

4. Bake in the preheated oven for 15-20 minutes, or until the salmon is cooked through and flakes easily with a fork.
5. Serve with lemon wedges on the side.

Spinach and Chickpea Salad

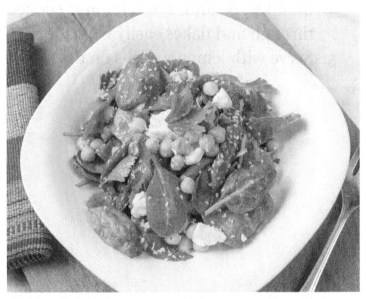

This salad is packed with fiber, protein, and vitamins. Spinach is rich in iron, calcium, and antioxidants, while chickpeas provide plant-based protein and fiber. This combination supports digestive health and helps maintain energy levels.

Nutritional Information (per serving):

- Calories: 250
- Protein: 10g
- Carbohydrates: 30g
- Dietary Fiber: 10g

- Sugars: 5g
- Fat: 10g
- Saturated Fat: 1.5g
- Sodium: 220mg

Ingredients:
- 4 cups fresh spinach leaves
- 1 can (15 oz) chickpeas, drained and rinsed
- 1 small red onion, thinly sliced
- 1 cucumber, chopped
- 1 avocado, diced
- 1/4 cup feta cheese, crumbled
- 2 tablespoons olive oil
- 1 tablespoon balsamic vinegar
- Salt and pepper to taste

Preparation Instructions:
1. In a large salad bowl, combine spinach, chickpeas, red onion, cucumber, and avocado.
2. In a small bowl, whisk together olive oil, balsamic vinegar, salt, and pepper.
3. Pour the dressing over the salad and toss to combine.
4. Sprinkle with feta cheese before serving.

Turkey and Avocado Wrap

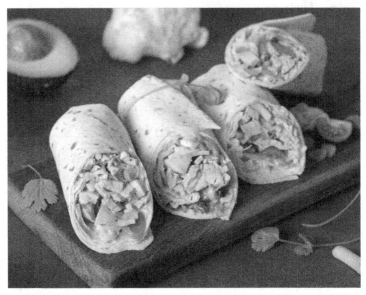

This wrap is a balanced meal providing lean protein from turkey, healthy fats from avocado, and fiber from whole-grain tortillas. It's great for maintaining muscle mass and providing sustained energy.

Nutritional Information (per serving):

- Calories: 300
- Protein: 20g
- Carbohydrates: 28g
- Dietary Fiber: 8g
- Sugars: 2g

- Fat: 12g
- Saturated Fat: 2g
- Sodium: 450mg

Ingredients:
- 4 whole-grain tortillas
- 8 slices of turkey breast
- 2 avocados, sliced
- 1 cup baby spinach
- 1 tomato, sliced
- 1/2 red onion, thinly sliced
- 2 tablespoons Greek yogurt
- 1 tablespoon lemon juice
- Salt and pepper to taste

Preparation Instructions:
1. In a small bowl, mix Greek yogurt with lemon juice, salt, and pepper to make a dressing.
2. Lay out the tortillas and spread the yogurt dressing evenly on each.
3. Layer the turkey slices, avocado, spinach, tomato, and red onion on the tortillas.
4. Roll up each tortilla tightly and slice in half before serving.

Lentil and Vegetable Soup

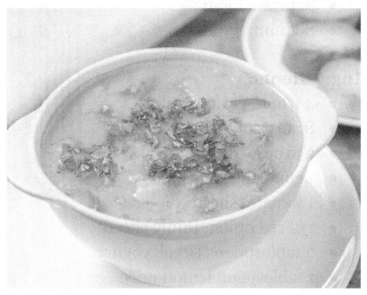

Lentils are a great source of plant-based protein and fiber, which help with digestion and maintaining stable blood sugar levels. This soup also provides a variety of vitamins and minerals from the mixed vegetables.

Nutritional Information (per serving):
- Calories: 250
- Protein: 14g
- Carbohydrates: 40g
- Dietary Fiber: 15g
- Sugars: 8g

- Fat: 4g
- Saturated Fat: 1g
- Sodium: 350mg

Ingredients:
- 1 cup lentils, rinsed
- 1 tablespoon olive oil
- 1 large onion, chopped
- 2 cloves garlic, minced
- 2 carrots, chopped
- 2 celery stalks, chopped
- 1 zucchini, chopped
- 1 can (14.5 oz) diced tomatoes
- 6 cups vegetable broth
- 1 teaspoon dried thyme
- 1 teaspoon dried basil
- Salt and pepper to taste

Preparation Instructions:
1. In a large pot, heat olive oil over medium heat. Add onion and garlic, sauté until soft.
2. Add carrots, celery, and zucchini, cook for 5-7 minutes.

3. Stir in lentils, diced tomatoes, vegetable broth, thyme, basil, salt, and pepper.
4. Bring to a boil, then reduce heat and simmer for 30-40 minutes, until lentils are tender.
5. Serve hot with a slice of whole-grain bread.

Meal Plans for Different Dietary Needs

Heart-Healthy Meal Plan

- **Breakfast:** Oatmeal topped with fresh berries, a handful of walnuts, and a drizzle of honey.
- **Mid-Morning Snack:** A small apple with a tablespoon of almond butter.
- **Lunch:** Spinach and chickpea salad with a whole-grain roll.
- **Afternoon Snack:** Carrot sticks with hummus.
- **Dinner:** Baked salmon with lemon and dill, served with steamed broccoli and quinoa.
- **Evening Snack:** Greek yogurt with a drizzle of honey and a sprinkle of chia seeds.

Diabetic-Friendly Meal Plan

- **Breakfast:** Scrambled eggs with spinach and a slice of whole-grain toast.

- **Mid-Morning Snack:** A small handful of almonds.
- **Lunch:** Grilled chicken salad with mixed greens, cherry tomatoes, cucumber, and a light vinaigrette.
- **Afternoon Snack:** Sliced bell peppers with guacamole.
- **Dinner:** Quinoa and vegetable stir-fry with tofu.
- **Evening Snack:** Cottage cheese with sliced strawberries.

Bone Health Meal Plan

- **Breakfast:** Greek yogurt parfait with granola and fresh blueberries.
- **Mid-Morning Snack:** A smoothie made with almond milk, spinach, banana, and a tablespoon of chia seeds.
- **Lunch:** Kale salad with grilled salmon, quinoa, and a lemon-tahini dressing.
- **Afternoon Snack:** A small piece of cheese with whole-grain crackers.

- **Dinner:** Baked chicken breast with roasted sweet potatoes and steamed green beans.
- **Evening Snack:** A glass of fortified orange juice.

Anti-Inflammatory Meal Plan

- **Breakfast:** Chia pudding made with almond milk, chia seeds, and fresh berries.
- **Mid-Morning Snack:** A small handful of walnuts.
- **Lunch:** Mixed greens salad with roasted vegetables, quinoa, and a turmeric dressing.
- **Afternoon Snack:** Sliced cucumber with hummus.
- **Dinner:** Grilled mackerel with a side of sautéed spinach and sweet potato wedges.
- **Evening Snack:** Herbal tea with a piece of dark chocolate.

Made in the USA
Monee, IL
17 September 2024